MW00932059

Cover design by ITP & Me

Edited by Alexis Gibson

First edition published in Australia through ITP & Me

ISBN: 1517347866

ISBN-13: 978-151734784 (KDP)

Medical Disclaimer:

Nothing in this book could or should ever substitute for qualified medical advice and care. Most things in the book are taken from my experience and the observations of those around me. Information is anecdotal unless otherwise referenced.

This book is for everyone who has lived with ITP,
and for Leigh, who lives with ITP through me.

Immune Thrombocytopenia

HOW DOES IT FEEL to be told that you have an unpredictable autoimmune disorder that will affect your blood's ability to clot and heal? How does it feel to be told the treatment will impair your immune system's ability to fight off infection, weaken your bones, and interfere with your reproductive organs?

How does it feel to be told at 22-years-old that you will not be able to conceive and deliver a child without an enormous amount of medical intervention, that the medication you need to manage the disorder will most likely, over a long period of time, affect your body's ability to regulate hormones, shut down your adrenal system and increase your risk of diabetes, heart disease and obesity? Oh, and also raise your stress levels, thin your skin, weaken your nails, affect your sleep, shorten your life span and weaken your eyes?

How does it feel to be told there is little to no information about your disorder; that every case is different and will most likely be compounded with a number of other autoimmune disorders as you age; that there is no long-term plan for the treatment of your disorder and all you can do is suppress your immune system and try to manage the side effects?

The answer to all these questions is this... Fine!

It feels fine because it will never happen to you!

That's what everyone thinks. That's what I thought; bad things happened to other people. I know it sounds like a cliché, but I really believed that I was indestructible. Chances are, though, if you're reading this book then it *has* happened to you, or someone you love.

The first time I heard that long speech, I was in shock. I thought to myself, 'Yes, yes, that's all very well and good for someone else, but none of that will happen to me,' even though, at that exact moment it was happening to me. 'I'm just hearing the worst case scenario,' I told myself. I was in complete shock when I was diagnosed with ITP. I felt great!

My story is similar to other stories I've heard from people with ITP: having ITP sounded terrible, but I thought mine would be the kind of ITP that went away. It wasn't.

I was diagnosed with ITP while I was on my lunch break from work. I went to my GP to get blood test results in a carefully planned lunch hour that would see me hurriedly eating sushi in the waiting room. I walked up to the reception desk, unaware that my phone (on silent) had three missed calls from my doctor telling me to head straight to the ER. I sat in the waiting room blissfully unaware, looking up at Finding Nemo on repeat on the television above the receptionist, dripping soy sauce artfully onto chicken teriyaki rolls. I had thirty five minutes until I needed to be back at work. There were two people ahead of me, and I was worried I would be late getting back to work.

When my doctor opened his door to call in his next patient, he noticed me sitting there. He told his patient that she needed to wait and ushered me quickly into the examination room. He had bad news.

I went straight back to work, picked up my bag, and had my boss drive me to the ER; the doctors at the hospital were expecting me, and I was admitted immediately. I spent a sleepless night in a hospital ward and was still awake to watch the sunrise the next morning. I lay there looking out the window scared of what was about to happen. My friends brought flowers that I couldn't keep because the patients in the ward were immune compromised. I was immune compromised. A few days later, I was officially diagnosed with ITP.

It took a long time for me to sit down to write this book. There were a few false starts, a number of other projects popped up, and most importantly, I could not shake the feeling that I had nothing to offer. I stayed quiet.

But over the last few years, I feel like the conversations around ITP has slowly become negative. The dialogue I see online now around ITP is sad. Patients are confused, disheartened with their treatments, feeling isolated and exhausted. The tone of the emails I receive has changed. What was once joy and excitement to find people to talk to about ITP is now frustration that there are still no answers. Haematologists have also been the target of online complaints, and it feels as though more and more patients are taking a passive approach to their health care.

Increasing awareness around ITP has coupled with the seriousness and sadness of having ITP. Last year alone there were a number of sudden and startling ITP deaths.

I understand the sentiment, I feel it sometimes too. Which is why I wanted to create something positive and cohesive, something that could be a reference book for people with chronic ITP and a guide for those newly diagnosed. Something that could contribute to a positive discussion about ITP with everything collected together in one place. After more than seven years living with ITP and more than three years running one of the most visited ITP blogs, I finally decided it was time to contribute.

So what do we know? We still don't know if genetics, culture, or nationality play a part in someone's susceptibly to ITP, but that could be changing. As you read this, doctors in Australia are collecting and analysing an International ITP Register, *A Disease Registry for Adults Diagnosed with Primary Immune Thrombocytopenia (ITP) in International Countries*. The register was started in 2013 and researchers will be collecting data until December 2016. I can't wait until the research is released. News like this is very exciting and worth sharing.

As ITP is a rare disease, most patients have never heard of it before they are diagnosed. They have never met another person with ITP, and their general doctor has perhaps never treated anyone with ITP before. A patient's family and friends also rarely have experience with ITP.

On top of that, everyone is different. There is no 'typical' ITP story. Even though we all have the same disorder, we are all going through something quite unique and personal. Chronic patients have different experiences to acute patients, and children are different again to adults. Meeting other people with ITP is not always that helpful - because your experience of the disorder is so different from others. Which is why this book does not focus on platelet counts, numbers, treatments, or the small details of my story. It's about everything else: it's about living with ITP, not treating ITP.

Inspired by my most popular article from ITP and Me, *The Seven Stages of ITP*, this book aims to examine and expand on those ideas while also including healing ideas and treatments, tips and advice for life (including how to ace a blood test). One of my aims here is to address our responsibility in educating those around us about ITP, and the best way to go about it. I have also included a few basic first aid tips and things I have picked up along the way.

Our perspective and attitude towards ITP is the number one thing that can instantly change our lives, and that is the point of this book. The more information there is for patients, doctors and families, the more we can remove fear for those who are new to this. The more you know, the easier it becomes.

26 things you might not know about ITP:

1. ITP is no longer called idiopathic thrombocytopenia purpura – the *idiopathic* and *purpura* part of the name have been dropped. It's just *immune* thrombocytopenia now, but the acronym is still ITP. Go figure. There are many doctors who don't know this, as the update happened after they left medical school. If you are looking for the most recent information online, make sure you use the new name.

2. ITP is not always simply caused by an overactive immune system as many people believe; it can also be caused by a dysfunctional immune system.

3. In some cases, ITP has been successfully cured with vitamin D treatments.

4. ITP is not always about platelet destruction. It is widely believed that ITP is caused by the destruction of platelets by the immune system, but for some of us it may also involve a lack of platelet production.

5. With ITP patients, the platelets you do have work well. The platelets in your system are often young, offering normal to advanced function.

6. You can get ITP from rubella (German measles), but it tends to correct itself soon after.

7. ITP is a potential side effect of some vaccines.

8. You can contract ITP from the MMR vaccine. The likelihood is about 1 in 40 000.

9. Acute ITP can occur after *any* viral infection.

10. Friends and family can donate platelets every two weeks (instead of whole blood every three months) via an apheresis machine.

11. ITP treatment is a growing investment industry with the apheresis equipment market expected to be worth $2, 885, 000, 000 by 2020.

12. ITP can lower your life expectancy by up to twenty years if you are not careful. This information came out of one small study.

13. Directly exposing a bruise to the vitamin D in sunshine will speed up the healing process.

14. ITP is twice as likely to occur in women as men.

15. Taking immune suppressants will affect the validity of your travel insurance policy.

16. You can decide which specialist you see.

17. You can choose your treatment plan for ITP.

18. You can drink alcohol if you have ITP and are responsible.

19. Every year there is an International ITP Conference held in America.

20. About 5% of all pregnancies will develop gestational thrombocytopenia. This low platelet count will normally correct itself soon after the birth.

21. Having ITP does not affect your chances of getting pregnant or having a baby.

22. ITP does impact your choices and decisions during the pregnancy and delivery of your child.

23. Having a low platelet count might limit your ability to have an epidural during a cesarian section.

24. Twenty percent of all ITP patients have *secondary ITP* as a result of another disease or autoimmune disorder.

25. Hashtags for people suffering from ITP are #itpawareness, #lowplatelets, #itpprobs, and #iknowaboutITP.

26. Alternative medicines and natural therapies do help.

History

IMMUNE THROMBOCYTOPENIA is the first ever recorded autoimmune disorder. ITP was discovered during an infamous experiment in the 1950s where doctors performed medical experiments on themselves and friends. To read about it now feels like a gothic horror novel.

The discovery of ITP involved dramatic experiments using blood plasma that helped form the modern basis of autoimmune theory. It would later be known as the Harrington-Hollingsworth experiment.

Dr Harrington's interest in immune thrombocytopenia began in 1945 when he was a twenty-two year old pre-medical student at Boston College. While studying, Harrington cared for a young woman with ITP. Under his care, the young women died from a severe haemorrhage. Five years later, in 1950, Dr. Harrington was receiving his haematology training at Washington University. There, he cared for another woman with severe bleeding, whose platelet count did not increase after a splenectomy.

During this time, it was not known what caused a low platelet count. There was a lively debate taking place in the medical community about the exact process of antibody interference with platelets: were they being destroyed or was platelet production being impaired? No one knew what caused ITP. Reports of mothers with ITP giving birth to babies with severe thrombocytopenia were starting to be shared and documented, leading some in the haematology community to suspect that there was a connection between mother and child. This connection suggested that the cause of platelet destruction was impairment rather than an external destructive force.

Harrington developed a hypothesis that platelet impairment was caused when platelets were destroyed by a plasma factor after they were produced by the bone marrow. The Harrington-Hollingsworth experiment was intended to establish the autoimmune nature of the blood disorder ITP. If Harrington was correct, the experiment would establish ITP's connection to the individual, not an outside virus or disease. He had an idea. All he needed to do was wait for a suitable candidate.

On a Sunday afternoon in 1950, a candidate appeared. Her blood was tested and showed a platelet count of five. At the moment before the experiment took place, Dr. Harrington had a platelet count of 250. To prove his theory, Harrington injected himself with the woman's blood and gave her an infusion of his blood.

While he waited for the woman's blood to transfuse through his veins, Harrington sat quietly reading a medical journal. The results were dramatic; he quickly reported flulike symptoms, and eighteen hours later he had marks on the ankles, petache on his skin, bleeding gums, and bruises up his legs.

Harrington's platelet count fell rapidly to nearly zero, and his colleagues insisted he remain in the hospital. It was five days before his platelet count recovered to normal. Meanwhile, the platelet count of the patient who had been injected with Harrington's blood did not change.

In spite of the clear dangers, this experiment was repeated with nine other ITP patients and several other volunteer physicians. Harrington reported doing the experiment on himself more than thirty times. Because the physicians' bodies did not produce the antibodies that destroyed platelets, their platelet count returned to normal within about 5 days. No one was permanently left with ITP, but nor was any ITP patient cured.

Harrington's work provided the first evidence for the production of antibodies against one's own tissues, and formed the initial basis for theories of autoimmune disease. The study was a milestone for understanding ITP, and led to ITP being the first documented autoimmune disease.

In the tradition of scientists infecting themselves with yellow fever, malaria, scarlet fever, and other dangerous diseases, this experiment could be described as heroic; however, these self-experiments may also be described as foolish with unnecessary risks. These days, experiments using human subjects must be reviewed by an impartial board of scientists, and unauthorised self-experimentation like Harrington's is no longer allowed.

We can say that we are wiser now than he was in 1950, but his results still stand as a landmark in the story of ITP. Harrington died in 1992 while repairing a generator outside his home, which had been without electricity and running water since Hurricane Andrew hit southern Florida.

Platelets. I've heard the word a thousand times.

I thought I knew all about them from high school science class. Platelets were just those tiny things that floated around in my blood and magically 'plugged up' leaks when I needed them, right? After my diagnosis, I learnt that there was a lot more to platelets than I originally thought.

First, where do they come from? Platelets are created by a larger cell in the body called a megakaryocyte. (No, I have never said that word out aloud.) Megakaryocytes are created from stem cells in the bone marrow. In pictures, they look like a pink fried egg, with a center yolk of cells and a fragmented white around it.

As a megakaryocyte matures, it fragments into platelets that are released into the blood. This fragmentation is triggered by the hormone thrombopoietin, which is secreted by the kidneys and liver. Without the liver producing this hormone, the megakaryocytes won't fragment into platelets.

Young platelets survive in the blood stream from between 7 to 10 days. During this time, platelets circulate the blood stream before finally being stored in the spleen for about 36 hours. When the body is injured and goes into repair mode, the spleen contracts and releases the platelets back into the blood stream.

When platelets are flowing through the blood stream, they are 'unactivated'. An unactivated platelet looks like a smooth round blood cell. When a platelet is activated, it grows sticky little arms that adhere to each other and to the injury site.

I've often wondered *how* a platelet could become activated. I won't presume to claim that I completely understand the process, but I do know that one way a platelet can become activated is in response to the presence of collagen. Collagen is found in almost every part of the body except the blood vessels. This means, for a platelet to come in contact with collagen, a blood vessel must be broken. Simple.

I am in awe of the thousand simple processes that happen inside the human body. When platelets are young, they absorb serotonin. Serotonin acts as vasoconstrictor, and this hormone remains in the plasma of the platelet until the platelets are activated at the onset of an injury. Once the activated platelet releases the serotonin, the blood vessels around the injury contract.

If a platelet lives its entire life (about 10 days) without becoming activated, it is the liver's job to remove it from the blood stream. As old platelets are removed, the liver secretes more thrombopoietin to trigger the megakaryocytes to fragment into more platelets. The life cycle is complete.

So how many platelets do you need? A 'normal' platelet count has a very wide range, and can be anywhere between 150 and 450 billion platelets per litre of blood. A person with a platelet count of 160 may be considered as healthy as a person with a platelet count of 420, it all depends on the individual. Any platelet count higher than 450 billion platelets indicates a potential health condition, and any platelets count lower than 150 billion platelets indicates a very different set of health problems.

Men and women often differ slightly in their 'normal' ranges.

Now that I better understand the cycle of platelets within my body, I feel like I am far better at taking care of my entire system. To properly take care of my platelets, I need to make sure I'm taking care of my bones, kidneys, liver and spleen. (Yes, I still have one, as much as I asked for it to be removed during some low months.)

I also now know that I can't always feel a low platelet count. In the early years of having ITP, I was convinced that I knew when my platelets were low because of how I felt, but my gut feeling wasn't always accurate. While I can mostly sense a low platelet count, I am sometimes very surprised and wrong.

Some ITP patients may never feel anything when their platelets fall while another feels everything. Most people can guess based on common symptoms of low platelet count: bruising easily and bleeding a lot. Others have frequent nosebleeds, petache rash, or bleeding gums. These symptoms are gross. They may also hurt and cause discomfort, pain and embarrassment. It's these symptoms that make ITP hard to hide.

Redness or blood in the corner of your eyes and dark, bruise-like circles under your eyes may also cause embarrassment. How many times have people said I look tired?

Lesser-known symptoms of a low platelet count are fatigue and pain in your joints. When my platelet count is low, I sometimes feel weak, unable to recover, and more likely to stop exercising.

Headaches are also a possible symptom of low platelets. Having a low platelet count can make you feel fragile, or weaker than you once were. It might make you feel different at the changes it has caused. Then again, you might not feel anything. Some people don't feel a low platelet count at all. So how is ITP diagnosed if there are often no symptoms at all?

ITP can present in a number of different ways. Patients will normally experience some level of tiredness or flulike symptoms but will often ignore this until it is accompanied by other warning signs such as bleeding, bruising, or the discovery of tiny red marks on the skin. A family doctor will then order a blood count; if the results show a low platelet count, you will be sent to

ER.

A bone marrow biopsy is usually done to rule out leukaemia or another bone marrow disorder, but this is not always necessary. A qualified haematologist will diagnose you with ITP. Currently, the only way to diagnose ITP is to rule out all alternatives, which means that ITP is diagnosed following a subnormal platelet count in the presence of normal bone marrow and in the absence of any other disease.

Dentists can also diagnose people with ITP based on bleeding in the gums. What might appear to be gum disease to the patient is something very different to a dentist.

The prevalence of ITP is approximately 9.5 cases per 100,000, although this number is an estimate. Like all autoimmune disorders, women (especially older women) are more likely than men to be diagnosed with ITP. In the 30 to 60-age range, more women than men have ITP, while in other age groups, roughly equal numbers of men and women are diagnosed with ITP (8). Although the connections between estrogen and ITP have been explored, there is no conclusive explanation for the sex bias in ITP.

It is interesting to note that pregnancy has been known to cause a number of autoimmune changes in women. For some, pregnancy can trigger the start of an autoimmune disorder, while in others it causes their disorder to go into remission. These cases have sparked an interest in the relationship between changes in autoimmune disorders and hormones (10).

Diagnosis & Denial

DENIAL IS ONE OF the most common defence mechanisms – it's easy and natural to pretend nothing is happening. It doesn't mean that you are insane or not coping. Denial often helps you get through what you need to and gives you time to process what is happening.

When I received my ITP diagnosis, I didn't even know I was in denial. In fact, I felt just the opposite. I told everyone about having ITP. I was happy to discuss it. I felt ok about my diagnosis. I thought it was funny. Denial.

Over the years, the story of my diagnosis has taken on a myth-like quality in my mind. Each time I remember my trip to the ER, it's faster and scarier than before. I think my platelets are lower every time I tell it.

But it actually all started long before that day. The truth is, I had been bruising badly for a long time, so much so that I'd became accustomed to the bruises. I thought of myself simply as someone who bruised easily. It must have been a long, slow platelet drop for me to become so casual about the bruises.

After finishing Uni I quickly set about planning a trip overseas. For a year, I worked full time and prepared for the eagerly awaited adventure – my first time out of Australia. In the months leading up to the trip, a retired nurse told me to 'get those bruises checked out.' I winked in reply and made a joke about being a delicate person. I was scared to go to the doctor so close to leaving the country. I knew if I went to the doctor before I left, there could only be two possible outcomes.

The first outcome was that the bruises meant nothing, I was just someone who bruised easily and a trip to the doctor was a waste of $65 that would have been better converted to pesos and spent on beers in a Mexican bar.

The second outcome was that my bruises meant that I was fatally ill and probably going to die from a terrible cancerous disease. In which case I would not be able to go on my holiday around the world and would die a loser that had never been out of the country. I wasn't going to let that happen. If these bruises were going to kill me, then I saw it as even more of a reason to go traveling.

It's weird to think about how dumb that sounds now. I wasn't the smartest little twenty-two year old but I left Australia for 3 months and had the most incredible time. I bruised while I traveled, but mostly everything was fine. I was exhausted but assumed it was jet lag. I was sore, but I was pushing myself and sleeping badly in hostel dorms. I walked everywhere with a backpack on and expected that I would need a lot of sleep. I though I had a bit of the flu, but I was staying out late in the cold. I felt sick, but I was in Mexico. Everything made perfect sense. I came home just in time to sleep through the Christmas holidays.

When I came back, I was still alive but tired and obviously unwell. I felt ready to go to the doctor and had more time to address healing if it was a bad outcome. (Yes, I was an idiot!) I went to the doctor for my results during my lunch break at work. It was a morning of missed calls and rushing to the bus after another overslept alarm. I worked all morning while my doctor tried to get through to me.

When he rushed me into the examination room with a worried look on his face, I assumed he was overreacting.

I actually hated this guy. He once refused to give me the morning-after pill on the grounds that my mother would be happier than I expected to have a grandchild. He told me I owed it to myself to think about how my whole family would feel about a new baby. *Eye roll*

Needless to say, I was wary of this guy's judgment. Since my diagnosis, I have learned that there are beautiful genius doctors who will make your life a dream. (I'll get to them later; this man was not one of them.) My doctor had already called the ER and pre-admitted me, like at the airport. 'You can't go back to work,' he said. I was to go to the ER immediately, with my files scrunched in my sweaty little hands. That's when I believed it might really be something serious.

In the ER, I smiled as I waited. Denial. I didn't call anyone, except my older sister because I needed help with the Medicare forms, and I knew she had a copy of mum's card in her wallet. Denial.

As tests continued, the doctors at the hospital became more confident each time they mentioned ITP as a possible diagnosis. I thought having ITP was quite interesting and told myself, 'If I'm going to get anything, it may as well be something different.' Denial.

In the beginning, I was the perfect patient. I did everything I was told: I set an alarm to take my medication, went to bed early, and went to every appointment. I nodded and said yes to everything. I went where I was sent, and I did what needed to be done. I responded reasonably well to medication, and I was incredibly compliant.

That's the thing about denial; normally you don't know you have it. I secretly thought I could do something to make my ITP go away. I told myself that if I was really 'good' I would be able to reverse it. I thought, 'I'm different from everyone else, so it will be different for me'.

In the beginning, I was unable to admit to myself that my ITP might last, and it wasn't for years that I realized ITP wasn't going away. I still get a shock every now and again, when I think about it. 'Oh gosh, is this still going on?'

It has been 7 years now, and it's still going on. ITP has certainly changed the way I live, but not all of those changes are bad; I am healthier and gentler to my body than I used to be. But I missed the first year because I was in denial – I barely remember it now. I was walking around in a fog.

Here's what I'd do differently if I could live that year again.

I would make more of an effort to find out which type of ITP I had. An ITP diagnosis falls into two categories, primary and secondary ITP. Primary ITP is characterized by peripheral platelet destruction, while in secondary ITP the platelet destruction is associated with another autoimmune disease, malignancy, infection, or another cause. The clinical association of ITP with other diseases is well recognized, although the prevalence of secondary ITP among patients with underlying diseases varies considerably from 1% to 60%, depending on the underlying disease. Most of the studies concerning secondary ITP are characterized by the underlying diseases but not the core issues of ITP (14).

Does it matter which kind of ITP you have if you still have ITP? It is the same disease no matter where it came from and no matter what the reason, right? Well, actually it does matter if you want to get to the heart of the problem. It is important to know if you are facing ITP on it's own or ITP related to something else. In a study, of 20 people diagnosed with secondary ITP, 9 had systemic lupus erythematosus, 7 had APL syndrome, 2 had Evan syndrome, and 2 had Hodgkin disease. There can be a lot of other things going on behind your ITP.

I would start tracking my platelet count from that first day. In the first few months after being diagnosed, I relied on doctors and hematologists to record and monitor my platelet counts. If I could go back in time, I would start recording my platelet numbers from that very first test. Keeping a close eye on the rise and fall of my platelet count was key to removing a lot of my fears and worries. Over a long period, patterns began to emerge, and I started to connect platelet drops with environmental factors in my life.

I would keep detailed notes, including my medication, any other illnesses, varying stress levels, and anything else that may be significant later. My notes might include whether I moved house, started a new job, or went on holiday.

These records have been handy when I need to consult quickly with a different doctor, or I'm on holiday and need to see other medical professionals and alternative therapists. I would also collect them for my own curiosity, to see how I am going. But I wish I had that first year. Doctors will ask questions like: What is your lowest count? How low where your platelets when you were on X amount of steroids, or when you had the flu?

I recommend Health Monitor's free Smartphone App for ITP patients; it was specifically designed for ITP patients and can help you easily track your platelet count.

I would celebrate the International ITP Awareness Day on the last Friday in September. Originally started in America, International ITP Awareness Day is quickly spreading around the world. A number of Australian ITP'ers I know get very excited about it. There is no official way to celebrate ITP Awareness Day apart from wearing purple, telling all your friends about ITP and maybe having a party. Mostly this is the day people plan to have walks and runs to raise money for ITP; a good day to donate to fundraising perhaps?

Knowing what I know now, I would spend some time (and money) overhauling my first aid kit. For a long time I simply 'made do' with the things I had.

Small cuts and abrasions need pressure and strength when you have ITP, my days of using cheap Band-Aids are over. I now buy tight, waterproof, fabric Band-Aids to help stop the bleeding faster. I keep a couple in my bag, wallet, car, and kitchen.

Ice packs are also my best friend. I finally brought a couple of nice soft gel packs to keep in my freezer. These are excellent for bumps, falls, and whacks to the head from the kitchen cupboards.

When I travel I take travel cold packs. These plastic ice packs are ideal for traveling because they don't need to be kept cold. Instead, they become cold through a chemical reaction that can be engaged by squeezing the pack at any time. There are many different brands available online.

If your child has ITP, most schools will allow ice packs to be kept around the school for easy access. Older children may wish to access ice packs without too many teachers standing in their way. Being able to get an ice pack on their own will help children feel more independent and confident about managing their ITP. Ask the school about this as part of an overall plan for ITP in the playground.

For a long time, I was tempted to buy bruise cream for the first aid kit. These creams normally contain arnica and are available over the counter in most pharmacies. I've used them a few times, and while they are aesthetically helpful, I no longer like to use them on my bruises. My bruises provide me with a lot of information about my ITP, and I prefer to watch and monitor my bruises, as these are the first indication of platelet changes.

I would buy a new toothbrush, a soft one – the best thing I did for my gums was to buy a soft bristle toothbrush. Brushing my teeth with a low platelet count usually ends with bleeding gums and a sore mouth. I go gently into the night.

I would find out my blood type. I know it now, but I didn't 7 years ago. I was always asked what my blood type was, and I couldn't answer. I needed it for health forms and my medical alert. It is good to find out as soon as possible.

It's also important to know your blood type in case you require a blood transfusion to treat your ITP. Not because you will need to tell your doctor, but because you might need to tell all your friends and family. As I waited for surgery, I found out that the blood bank was low in my type, prolonging the date of my surgery. I then pestered friends and family looking for people with O Positive. Now that I think about it, everyone needs to find out their blood type, regardless of ITP or not.

I would talk to my friends more about ITP. In the first few years, I underestimated the presence and impact of my ITP on those around me. My friends and family had never heard of ITP (accept the few friends I have who work in haematology departments - random). I knew everything about ITP and hated being the one responsible to educate everyone around me. I got sick of explaining ITP to people and started looking exhausted when people forgot what I had.

As an ITP patient, it is important to remember that it is not always about you. Friends and family will worry about you whether they tell you or not. Talking to friends about ITP will not only help them to understand you but help you understand them. Take care and be patient when people ask about ITP, it means they are interested in you.

I would read more about ITP. I have always kept up to date with the ITP research, but the information regarding ITP is changing all the time. Hopefully everything in this book will be out of date in a few years. If that happens, I will let you know. Searching the Internet provides a vast amount of information to sift through. While most of it is old or anecdotal, that doesn't mean we should stop looking.

Lifestyle & Guilt

AFTER A FEW MONTHS, when my ITP did not go away, my feelings started to change. That was when I started to feel guilty. The haematologists at my hospital said research indicated autoimmune disorders are likely a lifestyle disease. I thought this meant that ITP was brought on by something that the patient had done or failed to do, or a virus they caught. After I heard that, I started to panic. I caused this? I became convinced that I had given myself ITP because I was a bad/lazy/irresponsible person.

I would later learn that the term 'lifestyle disorder' does not have as literal meaning as the words suggest, but for a long time I thought I had done this to myself. A few people around me also believed I had done this to myself and were quick to point out all the ways that my lifestyle was probably a factor.

My mind went into overdrive. I searched for the cause, the day it all went wrong: day zero. I was convinced if I could trace my ITP back to the exact moment I got it, then I could reverse whatever I had done.

I looked at everything. Was it alcohol consumption? Had I drunk too much before or during my trip overseas? Logically I knew that alcohol consumption couldn't be the cause of ITP, as children and babies are diagnosed with ITP more frequently than adults, but that did not stop me from feeling guilty about it.

Was it stress? I hadn't felt stressed before I got sick, but I still didn't rule it out as a factor. Perhaps I was stressed and hadn't even known!

Was I a negative person? Did I complain too much? Did I stay out too late at night? Had I inhaled too many paint fumes at art school?

Was it a virus? I've only ever had the flu once in my life. It was a few months before I left to go on my trip to Mexico, and it was the sickest I've been in my life. It was a crippling kind of flu where your bones ache, and you can barely move except to shake out the sweat from your skin. I thought I was going to die, and people laughed at my ignorance of never having had the flu before.

It is important to note that no scientific paper claims to have solved the autoimmunity mystery. I have my own theory about where autoimmune disorders come from, but frankly, it sounds crazy and has something to do with killer Mother Nature's self-destruct mechanism. (My theory has yet to be blind tested and peer reviewed and, therefore, should only be referenced as a hypothesis.)

Turning our attention to all autoimmune disorders, might help us gain a better idea of what happens to patients with ITP. The fact that there are more cases of autoimmune disorders diagnosed every day is alarming.

During the past twenty years, a significant increase has been observed in the incidence of autoimmune disease worldwide. In 2011, the American Autoimmune Related Diseases Association published a paper on the cost burden to America from autoimmune disorders, citing more than 50 million Americans are affected by autoimmune disorders today.

Genetics are certainly a factor but they cannot be the whole picture. It normally takes a very long time for the human genetic pattern to change enough to register on a worldwide scale, requiring many generations to pass. Studies have therefore been focused on the environmental factors of a rapidly changing (lifestyle!!) and evolving civilization. An article, *A Potential Link Between Environmental Triggers and Autoimmunity*, discussed rapid changes in the world that our bodies are unable to keep up with. These disturbances included changes in our lifestyle, nutrition, diet and environment. These are likely the kinds of things we need to look at when searching for the source of autoimmune disorders. These are the lifestyle problems.

Guilt is a natural response when a person feels or believes they have compromised their standards of conduct or gone against their moral standard. Guilt appears whether it is true or not. Guilt is a natural sign of intelligence. It relates strongly to remorse and is a sign that the 'guilty' person is taking responsibility for their perceived failures.

During my first year with ITP, I felt guilty towards my body, like I had let it down – I just could not figure out how. Feeling guilty is incredibly destructive because it can lead you to compare yourself to those around you. As you try to pinpoint what you did to cause your ITP, you start to think about your actions in comparison to others. Had I drunk too much while traveling around Mexico? If I had, then how much did everyone else drink? Surely, I was not the drunkest woman in Mexico City – Was I? Why didn't something bad happen to everyone else? If I am guilty, then why aren't all those people guilty too? Guilt is a bad place for your mind to be.

Immediately after I was diagnosed with ITP, I stopped drinking alcohol. It was a funny time; I completely cut out one part of my life without looking at my diet, lifestyle, sleep, stress, or exercise habits. It didn't take long to realize that there was no change in how I felt or in my platelet count whether I drank or not. I had gone cold turkey and failed to look at my life as a whole.

Slowly, and I mean slowly, I started to make small changes that stuck. With each trip to the supermarket, my husband and I replaced much-loved items with healthier options. Peanut butter from the supermarket became peanut butter from the health food store; peanut butter from the health food store became fresh almond butter from the health food store. When I eventually stopped eating bread, there was no need to buy nut butter at all.

It wasn't immediate, but it was easy. It was a slow change, and I adjusted as I went. Almost 8 years later though, I can see how far I have come. Our home is almost always paleo, and we've removed chemicals and artificial flavours from our diet. We now read the packaging on everything.

We occasionally treat ourselves to bad food, but we do so knowingly and can factor it into a week's nutrition. We cut out all the extra hidden sugars in our food. Now we eat the occasional lolly, knowing we are eating sugar and being overwhelmed and giddy with the power of it.

Eating less sugar means we crave less salt as well. We have reset our palate and can taste the flavours of vegetables again; carrots and pumpkin are sweeter and broccoli is more delicious.

Our dietary changes were slow. We achieved great change by making very small consistent adjustments to our diet over years.

Every now and again, we slip off-plan for a while but we don't see it as a failure, just part of the process. Our logical, practical minds are constantly in competition with our emotions and animal instincts to stock up on fat and sugar. It's ok. Like a child, I need calm and consistent discipline.

My desire to change our diet, while having a great outcome, came from a negative motivation. I have guilt to thank for that. I blamed myself for everything that had happened. I was certain it was my fault and that I had been terrible to my body for a long time.

I haven't healed my autoimmune disorder through food like others, but I haven't really tried yet. I am in a place where I am healthy and happy and ITP doesn't bother me, except for the occasional flare up that my body handles well.

In terms of exercise, I have been very lucky. A while ago, I fell in love with going to ballet class. It's easy to exercise three times a week when it's something you completely enjoy. I practice at home, look at ballet movies on YouTube, and look forward to the next class. Dancing offers cardio, strength and conditioning, as well as stretching and posture correction. I am usually out of breath during class, always sore the following day, and sometimes the strings inside my ballet shoes leave bruises on my feet. I remind myself that if I didn't have ITP I would still hurt after exercise. Exercise isn't easy - that is the whole point.

I strongly recommend choosing a form of exercise where you need to pay upfront. You'll be less likely to cancel if you have already paid - and it's easier to say no to friends if you can say, 'I've already paid.'

I hope you have found something you love doing just as much as me. I believe that there is an exercise out there for everybody. Like love, you just have to keep looking. Something will eventually fit, and you will find that exercising stops being something you apathetically add to the end of a laborious list.

Did I cause this? I have thought long and hard about this, and the answer is probably. It is hard to hear and even harder to accept. Guilt, however temporary can quickly turn to anger.

Bleeding & Anger

THE ANGRIER I AM about having ITP, the worse my ITP become. Anger has only prolonged my disease but I still slip into it every now and again, I can't help it.

The angriest I have been about living with ITP was when I begun to miscarry. The experience was dangerous, scary, and maddening. It was the most extraordinary loss as both my future and my health fell apart. That is when having ITP was worse than I could imagine.

While it was happening, I looked at every blood disorder website for help, even searching the haemophilia foundation for information on bleeding disorders and miscarriage (which if you know anything about haemophilia, is hilarious). There was little information available. Everything I could find that was a little helpful was anecdotal information from online forums.

I remember when we arrived with the news at the haematology department – they all kind of flipped out. I stayed there all afternoon trying to figure out what was going on. My platelets had already fallen. My medication was altered. Everything needed to be monitored.

I understood the possibilities of miscarriage. I knew that it happened all the time, and I didn't believe that having ITP increased my chances of miscarriage or caused it in any way. There is no evidence to indicate that someone with ITP is more likely to miscarry than anyone else. But having ITP did affect everything. It complicated every decision that needed to be made and was an issue at every turn.

There is enough to handle while miscarrying. There is the devastation, the hormonal crash, the sadness and the pain, the cramps, the mess, the exhaustion, and the fact that your life keeps moving on. You need a few days to stop but you can't because things are snowballing around you. Other people's babies are being born; people are talking about kids around you and you are unable to sneeze without holding your guts in place. Having ITP meant that I was not allowed to do any of that on my own.

I stayed closer to home and even closer to my husband. I sort of moved into his office. I stopped making plans in case I was trapped while out of the house. I Googled easy ways to get to the ER. I carried my phone to the toilet and my medical records to the supermarket. I saved my blood type into the locked screen on my phone.

There were lots of doctors, lots of blood tests, lots of ultrasounds, lots of medication changes, and lots of plans that kept changing; so many blood tests and bruises on my arms and wrists.

Miscarriages go on for a very long time. They can go on for weeks. I didn't know this at the time.

I ended up needing surgery. To be able to have surgery, my medication was increased to get a higher platelet count and approval from the blood bank.

During it all, my health deteriorated. I was back to where I was when I was first diagnosed with ITP. It was totally fucked. The ramifications of this lasted longer than I could have imagined.

I went to my first yoga class 7 days after the surgery. It took 10 more days before I stopped bleeding. On the 12th day, I attempted 5 sit-ups. I was on high dose steroids for a long time, and I was angry for even longer.

Anger is a pretty intense physical response. If feels overwhelming, a hot face, sweaty palms, a raised heart beat. It takes over my mind.

When looking at anger objectively it can be seen as productive. Anger is often such a powerful reaction to ones' environment that it motives an individual to act and change their circumstance, respond to a threat, or leave a bad environment. Anger is a reaction. It is seen as one of the most primary responses a mature human can have and is valuable when dealing with survival. Anger mobilizes. (Note, I am not talking about violent anger or aggression here.)

Problems arise when people do not know what to do with their anger, when people do not know how best to express and process it.

Comparing your life to another person's life is the easiest way to feel angry, particularly if that person is a raging alcoholic with perfect liver function and zero autoimmune disorders. I have compared myself to smokers, drinkers, criminals, people who eat McDonald's, people who drink coke and take drugs, people who party hard, and those who are stressed at work. It wasn't pretty. I was angry. And it got me nowhere.

If you find yourself angry, chances are you are misdirecting your anger in a number of stupid ways. You may feel angry with your doctors, thinking that they let you down in some way. You may feel anger towards your family and friends, those who are closest to you and who are trying to help the most. You may be angry with yourself for having such a frustrating body, or for making stupid choices when you were young. (Yes, I ate a lot of microwaved food, too.)

As more than twice as many women than men have ITP, it makes sense to discuss how ITP can and does affect the ladies. There is not much information out there for women looking for help with ITP and heavy bleeding, or even much information about any bleeding disorder and lady troubles.

But there is a lot of research looks at ITP and pregnancy. In addition to women who already have ITP, there is also gestational thrombocytopenia that presents itself in 5% of all pregnancies in healthy women. The Platelet Disorder Support Association (PDSA) has a document for pregnancy with ITP. They say that:

'Many women with low platelets are concerned about having a family. A low platelet count does not prevent a woman from becoming pregnant or delivering a healthy baby. However, the situation does require special attention and close coordination between the woman's hematologist, obstetrician, and pediatrician. (15)'

Every ITP pregnancy is different and the key really is to be prepared for anything.

Mild thrombocytopenia, where a pregnant woman's platelets fall slightly during gestation, is quite common. For more information, read *How I Treat Thrombocytopenia in Pregnancy*, (16) in which the discussion includes the antenatal and perinatal management of both the mother and fetus. It's incredibly comprehensive, and I could not do it justice in this book. It is the best ITP pregnancy reading material I could find.

Miscarriage and the loss of a child during pregnancy is probably the worst, most private kind of grief a woman can go through. It's the kind of grieving where no one wants to touch you, where you look like a collapsed version of yourself, and suddenly you can't understand anything anyone is saying. At least that's what it felt like to me.

In any natural miscarriage with a healthy mother, there is always the threat of bleeding too much. For (the few) women with haemophilia, ITP or other bleeding disorders, there is an even greater threat of haemorrhage. Mostly, a miscarriage is an incredibly private experience, but not for a woman with ITP. With an ITP miscarriage, there are a lot of people involved, and you are not often alone.

If this has happened to you or a woman in your life, I'm sorry. Here is a little plan to help you get through it, along with all the other stuff they tell you to do, drink plenty of water. This sounds like something I would say if I had no clue, but water is really important. I drank more water than I ever thought I could. Abdominal and lower back pain is the most common symptom of miscarriage, to the point where I could not contract those muscles at all. I had to hold both my hands on my stomach to cough it hurt so much. I didn't even have the strength in my abs to do a number two (water). As my hormones started to crash, I found in the weeks after that I was covered in pimples (water). Drink water.

Then drink a big glass of red wine. I mean one of those glasses you get from Ikea that can hold half a bottle of red without looking offensive. Don't just drink the red wine because it is a cliché; drink it because it is a depressant. The alcohol will slow you down, help you sleep and bring a bit of stillness. Feel it. Go right in there and get all the tears out.

Keep taking care of yourself. I returned to exercise through yoga - this was for my mind and body. Tell the teacher you have a heavy period but want to try and participate or, if you feel comfortable with your teacher, tell them you have miscarried. Yoga will wake up your the body again and get it moving. This will also help with back pain, abdominal soreness, and tightness in your hips. If you needed a D & C, it will also help gently reintroduce your pelvic floor muscles to exercise, as they may have been stretched during surgery. I bravely told my teacher what was happening, and she was excellent. I think yoga teachers actually love that shit.

Stop eating chocolate and bad food. There is nothing worse than waking up from the miscarriage coma and realising you also got heaps fat. It might sound like a shallow thing to be concerned about, but it can really prolong the sadness if you do not recognise yourself in the mirror. Your sense of self is vital at this time.

Stop Googling 'ITP and miscarriage' and go to bed. You could read forever and still be conflicted between the stories you find online. If you search long enough, you will find everything.

Dealing with anger can be very difficult. I did not realise just how angry I was. Often most of my anger was directed at the ITP itself, which is stupid since it is part of my body. I needed to get over it. Once I realized my anger needed action I moved very quickly from anger into my favourite stage of life with a chronic illness: *bargaining*.

Alternative Therapy & Bargaining

I WAS PETRIFIED THE first time I (knowingly) traveled overseas with ITP. I had read a number of travel insurance policies which quite clearly stated that anyone currently taking immune suppressant medication is in no way covered by their policy.

Adding to my worries about leaving the country was that Australia also has a wonderful health system. I felt nervous leaving the safety and security of a system that cares for me for free, and doctors that knew me by name. But I wanted to leave the country again. I wanted to keep traveling and doing all the things I used to do, so I did something crazy and went anyway. I traveled to Fiji with my mum, without any travel insurance. For six days. It was one of the scariest things I've done.

I have a friend who works for a travel insurance company. She knows all the horror stories. One particular story she told me has stuck in my mind about a man who traveled around the world without travel insurance. Somewhere in Southeast Asia, he was in a scooter/motorbike accident and ended up breaking his spine. A C4 break. He lost all movement below his neck. As if that wasn't tragic enough, his family couldn't afford to bring him home; he needed a special medical aircraft to transport him home, and it would cost millions of dollars.

He was stuck overseas indefinitely.

I sometimes wonder if he ever got home or if he is still there now, trapped in paralyzed nothingness. This man was on my mind as I got onto the plane. We boarded a plane from Sydney, flying eight hours to a developing nation for a weeklong holiday. I thought of him as we soared through the clouds. I made a mental note not to drive a scooter or motorbike anywhere. Needless to say, I also didn't drink the water.

The trip was wonderful, and everything was fine. When I came home, I wrote about my journey and posted in online. A few weeks later, I received an email from a woman who read my story. She too had ITP and was interested in traveling overseas. She told me that she was able to get travel insurance by registering her illness with the insurance provider and talking at length with someone on the phone about it. Once the finer details were explained and negotiated, she was able to get custom coverage. I was thrilled, as my husband and I wanted to travel to Indonesia and later Thailand and Vietnam.

In the lead up to our next holiday, I gave my insurance company a call and we started negotiating. Could I be covered for this even though I wasn't covered for this? Could I make my own plan? What if I was in a car accident? What if my bags were stolen, and, therefore, my medication was gone? I couldn't have everything, but I didn't have to give it all up. I customized my plan and traveled Indonesia and Thailand with almost full coverage. I was learning how to bargain.

Bargaining is the hopeful stage, the form of attempting to negotiate different or better terms of an agreement. It requires both sides to be rational and open to discussion. It does work with travel insurance companies, but it doesn't work with your immune system. When it comes to bargaining and negotiating over travel insurance, there can be progress made with the person on the other end of the line. With your own body, it's a little trickier.

Mostly, bargaining looks like late night Googling of obscure cures for ITP. Bargaining is the process by which you are convinced you can exchange something (in your life) for your health back. Bargaining might sound stupid to others, but it's important to remember that the process of bargaining, deciding what you would and would not give up in return for your health, is actually an incredibly positive process.

Bargaining is a form of hope. It is not to be treated lightly or laughed at. 'If I do X then maybe I will get Y, or maybe Z will happen'. If I give up chocolate, can I have my immune system back?

While bargaining can often be confused with denial, the difference is that bargaining offers the ITP patient a sense of agency and control. Bargaining is my favorite stage for just that reason – it offers hope.

I am very good at bargaining. I think that this is the stage I've spent the most time in. I often told myself that I am just one simple step away from solving the whole ITP/Autoimmune mystery. I also love that I secretly feel like a 1920's detective at this stage.

I've bargained gluten one month and dairy the next. I've decided that I'll never drink alcohol/coffee/caffeine ever again, and that I'll meditate every day and sacrifice sleeping in for a cure. I've promised to practice new breathing techniques and brought lots of different kinds of tea.

You may or may not sound crazy at this point. Your friends and family probably can't keep up with all the changes you are making in your life. I'm sure mine didn't.

Bargaining can be fun and hopeful, but it is rarely a sustainable frame of mind (otherwise it would be the last stage, not the fourth – obviously!). Most people get over bargaining naturally, as they realize all their efforts are too short term, too impulsive.

Bargaining small items to no avail is a wonderful way of realizing that healing is going to need a longer, more holistic and planned approach. Not just a quick fix with new tea - healing needs a whole life approach. Mind and body and alcohol and chocolate.

For me, I realized that I needed to incorporate alternative medicine into my world and not just rely on western medicine. I was eating healthily and exercising, but I needed to do more. I need to change my head and my mind as well as my body. Understanding alternative medicine can open new areas of knowledge about your ITP.

Alternative therapies are a great way to look at your whole life. Alternative therapies can be a blessing and a curse for those with bleeding disorders. They may be helpful, but they are not to be treated lightly or kept in secret from your doctors. You may find that your doctor warns you away from trying non-western treatments. I have found that this skepticism is based in an understanding of the detrimental effects alternative medicines can have. A doctor recently disclosed to me that she had a patient who almost bleed to death on the operating table because the patient had failed to disclose her keen consumption of Chinese herbs. I can't stress enough the importance of chatting with your doctor about what you would like to try. If your doctor seems to be very closed minded and dogmatically against alternative medicine, find a doctor who isn't.

Below, I have compiled a list of the most popular alternative therapies for people with ITP, and some common problems you might face while using them.

Yoga. The word yoga has come to mean 'a type of low-impact physical exercise,' but yoga has a long and rich history. Yoga is an ancient practice that originated in India. It includes eight limbs of yoga practice: *yama*, ethical standards for living and integrity, focusing on behavior; *niyama*, self-discipline and spiritual observances; *asana,* the postures practices in yoga, the limb of yoga most people are familiar with; *pranayama*, controlled breath, helps you recognize the connection between the breath, mind, and emotions; *pratyahara*, the practice of withdrawal to observe your external cravings and habits; *dharana*, focused contemplation; *dhyana*, meditation; and *samadhi,* ecstasy and the connection to divine. Joy fulfillment and freedom.

Yoga is a whole life approach to healing.

I have yet to find evidence of any adverse effects of yoga on patients with ITP. As it is a low-impact activity, there is little chance of bruising and injury, although yoga positions involving inversions (where your heart is lower than your heart) make some people light headed or dizzy.

Chinese herbs. Chinese herbs have been used for centuries; recipes for Chinese herbal remedies have been found in sealed tombs dating back to 168 BC. Chinese herbs continue to be very popular and widely used in both China and the western world. There are roughly 13,000 medicinals used in China. They can be taken as powders, tablets, or most commonly brewed into tea.

Using Chinese herbs is a long-term approach to healing. Treatments need to be continued over a long period, and it can take months or years to notice a change. This can make the use of Chinese herbs expensive. While appointments with herbalists may be covered by private health insurance, the herbs themselves rarely are.

Chinese herbs contain active ingredients that may alter or interfere with your other medications. Their use is not benign, and you should only undertake this treatment under the supervision of a knowledgeable herbalist, with your GP and haematologist. These herbs have active ingredients with real effects.

Acupuncture. Acupuncture is a sub-category of Chinese traditional medicine. Treatments involve the insertion of small needles along meridian lines of the body. These meridians are believed to be channels of energy where blockages can causes health problems. Acupuncture needles relieve these blockages.

While the use of acupuncture dates back to the first century, the Communist Party actively encouraged its use after Chairman Mao's rise to power. Farmers were trained to be rural doctors (called 'barefoot doctors') but lacked the resources to treat patients with contemporary medicine. Instead, they often turned to traditional treatments like acupuncture because they were cheap, acceptable to the Chinese, and used the skills already familiar to those in the countryside (17).

The perceived risk with acupuncture and ITP is that the patient will bleed or bruise, however, the needles are so thin it is unlikely. I have never had a bruise from acupuncture.

Ayurvedic medicine. Ayurvedic medicine is an ancient Hindu healing practice. The treatments included in this field are incredibly varied, and I am doing it no justice by trying to summarize it into a paragraph.

At its most basic, Ayurvedic medicine emphasizes balance and considers suppressing natural urges to be unhealthy. Ayurvedic doctors regard physical existence, mental existence, and personality as a unit, with each element influencing the others. I love the mental and spiritual aspect of this practice. I have only just started to touch the surface with sleep patterns, oil pulling and meditation.

Meditation. Studies have shown that meditation has both short- and long-term effects on various perceptual faculties. Herbert Benson, founder of the Mind-Body Medical Institute (which is affiliated with Harvard University and several Boston hospitals), reports that meditation induces a variety of biochemical and physical changes in the body collectively referred to as the "relaxation response."

There are many different types of meditation, including guided visualizations. Many religious practices also include some form of meditation. Research on the processes and effects of meditation is a growing subfield of neurological research. The most well studied form of meditation is *transcendental meditation,* which has been shown to help lower blood pressure. The practice involves the use of a mantra and is practiced for 15–20 minutes twice per day while sitting with the eyes closed.

Affirmations. Affirmations, or affirmative prayers are currently trendy thanks to popularization by famous people like Oprah, the Spirit Warrior, and Louise Hay. The practice involves focusing on a positive outcome rather than the negative situation. The self-help community has promoted the use of affirmations as a method to gather wealth and get a better job, but I feel it has been overlooked for dealing with illness. Affirmations can help you focus on the great things your body can do and help put ITP in perspective. For example, '*Yes I have ITP and bruise a lot but I also have a heart that pumps my blood around my body to cause such bruises. If I didn't then I would be dead *Smile at self in the mirror**'

Reiki. Reiki was developed in the 1920's by the Japanese Buddhist, Miako Usui. The practice is based on qi, which practitioners say is a universal life force, and involves "laying on of hands" by a practitioner to cause changes in the energy field of affected body parts. There is currently no scientific evidence that qi exists or that Reiki is effective at treating medical conditions. The positive benefits people feel after a Reiki treatment may be the result of spending time with the practitioner in a calm setting. I have had it, and it feels nice.

Applied kinesiology. Applied kinesiology was developed by a chiropractor. The essential premise of this practice is that every organ dysfunction is accompanied by weakness in a specific corresponding muscle in what is termed the "viscerosomatic relationship". Applied Kinesiology addresses all aspects of health, including mental, structural, and chemical elements.

I have had a number of kinesiology sessions and have loved each one. I must admit I sometimes forget a lot of the follow-up exercises, but I've never regretted a session. See my 'Favorite Things' in the back for details of a wonderful Sydney based Kinesiologist.

Naturopathy. Naturopathy is something I have yet to try. When I started to read up about it, I found that a lot of the fundamental ideas of naturopathic practice are simply common sense; the practice aims to prevent illness through stress reduction, and changes to diet and lifestyle.

It is, however, the rejection of evidenced-based medicine that can make naturopathy dangerous to ITP patients. I would recommend doing a lot of research about naturopathy, and talking to your doctor before pursuing it seriously.

Aromatherapy. Aromatherapy is a plant-based therapy and has been used for over 6,000 years. The main idea of aromatherapy is that the chemical (aromatic) compounds in plants can heal when they are inhaled or applied to the body. One example is the use of lavender oil to treat burns, and essential oils have been used to treat skin infections, pain, anxiety, and depression. Many plants have active ingredients, and aromatherapy is best administered by a professional.

Qigong. Qigong is a Chinese practice that aligns breath with movements and exercise, *qigong* is often called *moving meditation.* As a healing practice, there is little evidence that it can heal disease; however, it is an excellent way to spend time, relax, slow down, release stress and get in touch with your body. Perhaps that is how you heal disease after all.

Isolation & Depression

A WHILE AGO, after living for a long time with ITP, I found myself at home with the whole place to myself. My husband was out for the night and wouldn't be home for a while. I slipped into a nice kind of relaxing were I get important things done while doing a bit of dancing. After a long soak in the bathtub and half a glass of red wine, I set myself up in the lounge room to take advantage of the extra space and quiet.

I was having an art exhibition in a few weeks and wanted to get started on framing the artworks. I had brought a few new frames and started pulling them apart, cleaning the large pieces of glass. I wiped each pane of glass with anti-static cloths and leant them carefully against the wall, out of the way then went into the kitchen to make tea.

As I walked out of the room into the kitchen, a piece of glass slipped silently down the wall and onto the floor, laying invisibly on the rug in the hallway. You can see where this is going.

I strolled casually back into the lounge room and stepped straight into the centre of the sheet of glass. With the full commitment of my weight right on the middle, I smashed the pane to pieces and I cut a deep slice down the arch of my foot.

I still feel weak just thinking about it. While I am writing this, my mouth is watering, and the bottoms of my feet feel all tingly.

Blood went everywhere. I hobbled to the kitchen sink and clutched my foot to my chest. I was stuck. Blood dripped gothically over the floorboards and soaked into my clothes. I didn't know what to do. I was in that strange frame of mind where I had no perspective. Was this a big deal? I couldn't tell. Normally when two people look at a wound together, they can give each other an idea of how much to freak out. I didn't have that; all I saw was blood and felt such a hot burning in my foot I knew I couldn't walk. My phone was in the bedroom.

I sat there in shock. I bound my foot and waited for the bleeding to stop and my adrenaline to run down. When I could finally think, I crawled to my phone. Instead of calling the ambulance, I called my friend just to talk to someone. I wasn't alone. I don't think I even mentioned what had happened. I just chatted away and instantly felt better.

Thinking back, I don't think the cut was that bad. I didn't need stitches and could walk with a little hobble the next day. But it was the isolation, the loneliness, that rattled me. What if I died in my house, bleeding out on my kitchen floor before anyone could do anything? I was spooked. Since that moment, I've thought differently about medical alerts and having first aid information somewhere on my body.

Today, I have an emergency alert in my phone and have my details where people can read them, even when the phone is locked. Another option is a necklace or bracelet, which could work for a younger child who doesn't have a phone or someone who likes to have their information closer to them.

Looking at my phone, I feel safer knowing that everything is there for people to read. My screen saver has all my medical details saved on it.

These medical notes also sometimes catch my friend's attention as we sit drinking coffee, and they remember to ask how I am doing. It's a nice conversation starter and an easy way to let people know you are unwell.

I have also found that sometimes when I tell people about having ITP, they might give me a small cold nod and change the conversation. Those same people are later surprised to see I have a medical alert on my phone about ITP. I think it helps them understand that ITP is something I live with and think about every day. The medical alert makes it more real.

Feeling sad about ITP is a common occurrence for me. This depression can come on at any time, but for me it tends to arrive straight after the bargaining phase when I realise all my efforts have been a waste of time. It sends me to my room to throw myself (softly) down on the bed. In this moment, I don't want to try anything new. Any well meaning suggestion can be infuriating and help in any form can feel like an insult. I want to whine and wallow and feel sorry for myself. Depression is a bad place to be for too long.

This is the point when I feel like everyone is different from me. This is the moment when it seems like no one understands. Whether it is true or not, it feels like everyone around me is sick of hearing about my illness; that life has moved on while I'm still dealing with it.

This feeling doesn't last long. It comes in a wave and then eventually washes away. I also tend to get bored of being depressed quite quickly as no one wants to hang out with a grumpy loser.

This feeling shouldn't last too long, but if it does, think about seeking medical advice to process how you're feeling. Talking to professionals does help. Humans are safer, happier, and live longer when connected through a social life. Loneliness is meant to feel so bad that we make an effort to return to our people (I think). When people feel loneliness or isolation, they seek out warmth in ways like hot showers, warm drinks, tea, and staying in bed. Temporarily these things will help, but loneliness feels bad so you don't hang out in a depression forever.

I am very lucky to be involved in the ITP community. In being so, I often get to read other's ITP stories, chat with patients, and answer emails from people who are going through the same experience as me. It's incredible how many messages I get every week from people who are just happy to have found my website. These people felt isolated and confused for a long time before they managed to find like-minded people sharing the same journey.

Lucky we now have a International ITP Awareness Day. I was pretty excited when I found out about it, even if it is currently just in America. The last Friday of September is International ITP Awareness Day and in some places *Sport Purple for Platelets Day*. There is not a lot that happens on International ITP day but it gets bigger every year. You will also see ITP appear in social media and online a little, which is nice because it doesn't happen often.

International ITP day is a great day to start a conversation about ITP, and that seems to be the intention. It's not 'Cure ITP Day' or 'World ITP Research Day,' it's just about awareness. You could use ITP Awareness Day to tell one person, 'Oh, today is International ITP Awareness day,' and have them ask, 'Oh, what is that?' It starts a conversation that might not be easily brought up. It is also a reminder for friends and family to check in with the ITP patients they know.

It is hard to talk about hard things.

There is no special formula for talking to friends and family about being ill, and everyone is different. I have noticed that some people find it debilitating to ask for help, while others have no problem reaching out. No awards for perception here.

If your finding it difficult to talk to friends, it helps to realise what friends can and cannot do for you, and having realistic expectations of those around you. Identify what you actually want from your support people and then figure out how to get it, instead of just being sad and feeling depressed without any idea of how to make it better. Expecting people to constantly hug you and tell you they will walk you safely through life can put unreasonable expectations on your friends and family, especially if they think you want them to leave you alone. Do you want your friends to treat you like a sick person? Do you always act like a sick person in front of them? Not expecting too much of friends it important – they can only do so much to help you.

My understanding of ITP's affect on those around me was made clear when a good friend of mine published this post on my blog. Below is an excerpt:

My dearest friend has ITP. Her platelets fluctuate as do her doses of medication, access to good and bad information, her levels of being tired and in turn her mood. Each day that she wakes up she has ITP, and it isn't going away anytime soon. Meanwhile I go about my business, working, moving houses, seeing friends, working on different projects, all with my (for now) reasonably healthy body to take for granted. I wonder about my friend often. I wonder if she has been to the doctor lately.

I wonder what her blood count is, I wonder how much prednisone she is on, I wonder how much she wonders about it all. I see her posts pop up on her blog about living with ITP, and it reminds me, sometimes shocks me, that she is still living with ITP. I say shocking because often when shit things happen in your life you buckle up, breathe in, and try your best to move through them and come out the other side. We have all done this — buckled up, heard the bad news, cried and let the event finally pass. But this one isn't going to go away. Each day she continues to wake up with ITP.

My wondering has led me to ponder a couple of questions. How often should you ask your ITP suffering friend how they are doing, not wanting them to not feel alone and forgotten in it? How much do you allow them to remember and how much do you help them forget?

I thought the last sentence was perfect, as it is something I battle with myself: how much do I want to remember I have ITP and how much do I want to forget?

Depression and isolation are a common theme I see when patients reach out. They almost never know another person with ITP and have nothing to compare their own experiences to. Running a website about ITP has given me wonderful insight into common complaints and impacts. I also get many emails from patients wishing to discuss the impact ITP has had on their lives and how it has affected me. AS you may not have the time to start a whole website, I'll just share them here.

The most commonly mentioned issues are fatigue, fear and misunderstanding. Fatigue is a tricky one for people with ITP; as with many autoimmune disorders, patients often feel well enough to realise how bored they are. I know I need a great deal of sleep, particularly after exercising, but sometimes throughout the day I just can't seem to get ahead.

Not having enough energy to do everything, while having enough energy to look ok, is confusing and frustrating for others. People mention, 'Oh you don't look too bad today, you must be fixed!'

Fear is hard too, as it's not something people talk about very often. I find that ITP has increased how afraid I am of many things. For a long time after I was initially diagnosed, I was scared to walk up and down busy staircases, like those at airports and train stations. When I've tried to talk about fear, I found the first response people have is to tell you not to worry. 'That's silly', 'That will never happen', 'Just try to forget about that', or 'You're being too paranoid' are common responses. None of these responses do anything to address the things I'm genuinely worried about. People try to talk my worries away, make them disappear by belittling them. All that happens is I am discouraged from further talking about my fears as people try to trivialize them to make me feel better, so I stop telling people.

Misunderstanding is also hard. It can lead me to not wanting to talk about ITP. Some people think it's contagious. Or they think it's not a big deal.

Even with all of these issues, chatting about ITP with others is a great way to gain perspective and do a little reflection on just how good your life might be. As the only person in your social circle who has ITP, consider the effect your silence has on everyone. The more you talk about ITP, the more the whole world will know about it.

Bruises & Reflection

REFLECTION ALWAYS GETS me thinking and wanting to talk to others. During this time, I want to compare notes with other ITP people, ask questions and figure out what's going on. I want to look over past medical records, old platelet counts, and see how far I have come. I've been in and out of all these stages over the years, and my initial reflection stage led me to start the blog in 2012.

I'm always thinking about how I've been changed by ITP, and how my perception of the disorder has grown and developed over the years. In the beginning, I took ITP very seriously, and I had very strong ideas about what having ITP meant. Now, I am a lot more relaxed and at ease with it all. I am thankful that I have learnt so much, and I feel more in control of my health than ever. I feel like I am almost healed.

It was almost a year after my partner proposed to me, that we were married. It was exciting and weird and not something I ever thought we would do, yet there we were planning a wedding.

When it came to the dress, I knew exactly what I wanted – To cover up. I even made sure I had a long sleeve jacket to cover small elbow bruises made by blood tests in the weeks leading up to the wedding. It was important for me that bruises and ITP weren't in my photos or on anyone else's mind.

I organised to chat with a makeup artist in the months before the wedding and went to great lengths to learn the best way to cover up bruises. I learned that I needed to cover different coloured bruises with different shades of corrective concealer, and I felt quite empowered to know how to make them go away.

As the day grew closer, preparations intensified. I was so stressed about the wedding that I was sure I would make myself too sick to even attend. Which stressed me out further. It was a hard time.

In the end, I had one visible bruise, on the top of my foot. No one in the whole world would have noticed it, but I saw it in the photos. Our photographer simply Photoshopped it out. Gone.

During the night, as I danced outside under the fairy lights, I was bitten by a mosquito – a tiny little bite I felt nip at the back of my hip. It was itchy the whole night. A day later, near my hip there was a blue-black bruise larger than the side of my new husband's palm. But the wedding was over, and no one saw. I was able to hide ITP from my wedding. The bruise on my back stuck around for our whole honeymoon though.

What I've realised is that ITP can be hard to hide even when you want to. Sometimes it's just a little too public. I've learned that sometimes people with ITP just look like junkies. From the outside, the distinction between junkie and ITP patient is pretty damn small. I don't have anything against junkies; they have always got funny stories and have brightened the character cast of *Orange is the New Black* for three great seasons now. I digress. Looking like a junkie is just another fact of ITP that people don't often talk about.

Reasons you might look like a junkie are as follows: bruises, a red rashes, track marks, tired eyes, mood swings, late nights, nausea, fragile skin, liver damage, confusion and finally, paranoia - thinking every sharp corner is out to get you!

Ok, so I can't help you with the paranoia. I find that most of the time, when people think everything is out to get them, it's normally true. But for the rest, here are a few ideas to help you hide it when you need.

Bruises. Rest your bruise. If you have knocked yourself and you know it, the best thing to do is rest the area. Yes, I know resting is hard and lame, and no one really does it. So let's move onto the next one, ice.

Apply a cold pack. Blood runs faster when it is warm. If you can get ice onto your bruise as soon as possible, it will not only help heal the bruise but will keep it smaller to begin with. Any cold pack, ice, or bag of peas will help the healing process. This approach also requires you to know that a bruise is coming.

Bruises also respond well to compression. Keep the pressure on; bandage or tape the bruise. What you are doing is applying pressure to a wound to stop the internal bleeding. It is exactly the same thing for bruises as it is for cuts; most of us seem to forget that a bruise is caused by a rupture inside us that needs pressure to be applied. A bruise is a wound too.

Massage the area. After a bruise has blossomed, move those muscles. A bruise is caused by blood gathering and bleeding under the skin. Moving your muscles and getting your lymphatic system moving is a good way to move that blood around so it can drain away. When massaging a bruise, you need to be very gentle. It is not meant to hurt. Gentle walking is another way to get that blood under the skin moving.

Eat an orange. Increase your intake of Vitamin C. You probably eat very healthy anyway and telling you to take more vitamin C is stupid because of course you eat enough vitamin C, right? Get the oranges.

Get yourself into the sunshine. When hemoglobin (blood product) breaks down, it produces bilirubin. Bilirubin is what causes that yellowish colour around a bruise as it fades. The good news is that vitamin D in sunlight heals and breaks down bilirubin. Magic! If possible, expose the bruise to about 10 to 15 minutes of sunlight to accelerate the breakdown of the bilirubin. It really works.

Arnica. While I wanted to include Arnica on this list, I still have many questions about how one might actually 'take' it. Arnica is a naturally occurring flower that has been used for centuries in the healing of bruises. With arnica, there is a risk of toxicity, which I believe is why so many people online recommend taking it in tablets, as a gel, or using creams. The only form I could find for taking arnica safely was in commercially produced tablets, which defeats the purpose of using something natural, doesn't it? Which brings me to bruise creams and ointments: mostly they just contain arnica. These are intended to be applied directly to the bruise and not taken internally.

If you are still struggling for a quick fix, you could always apply a few leeches. Not recommended.

Track marks. Track marks are those long messy bruises you can get in the crook of your elbow after a blood test. To control track marks, it's important to understand where the bruise (blood) is coming from. When you get a blood test, the needle will leave two holes in your body, one in the surface of your skin where it enters your body and the second in the surface of your vein where it enters your blood stream. It might sound obvious but the bruise doesn't appear from the hole in the surface of your skin, it comes from the hole in your vein. Most of us only see the tiny little hole in our elbow, and apply pressure to that, but the hole you need to apply pressure to is under the surface of your skin, in that little vein that just got broken into.

So when the nurse tells me to apply pressure after a blood test, *I actually press*. After the test is over, don't use your arm for a few hours. I mean it – don't use it. Don't pick up your purse, carry shopping bags, or start making crafts. Just leave it still.

Skin. When it comes to your skin, two elements are at play. First, your medication might be drying your skin, leaving it thin, fragile, and splotchy looking. Second, there is the fact that if I scratch my skin, I get a big stupid lump of dried blood on my face and red blotchy skin. Pimples bleed, scratches bleed, mosquito bites bleed – everything bleeds. My skin often gets cracked and gross. The best solution is to take good care of your skin in the first place. Moisturise, drink plenty of water, buy some lotion, and choose makeup carefully.

Tired Eyes. My eyes sometimes get red and puffy. Apart from actually getting lots of sleep (which is the best technique I can recommend), I can also suggest lying when people ask you why you look tired. I tell people I went out late last night, or that I'm secretly a rockstar. Alternatively, you could tell them about having ITP.

Irritability, confusion, and mood swings. Most medications needed to treat ITP are mood alterers, but you are also on the ups and downs of having ITP. One day I'm embracing the disorder and getting used to having it and then boom, something cracks me, and I'm shitty and annoyed again that I have to deal with it. Fighting with my weird brain is a huge problem.

Liver Damage. Liver damage is a tricky one. Chronic medication users always run the risk of liver damage. Be good to your liver, especially with all the other crap it has to process. This includes food, exercise, nutrition and other drugs. Try not to get too drunk, because otherwise you really will look a lot like a junkie.

Understanding & Acceptance

'BOY! YOUR PLATELETS get low,' said my haematologist, sitting in a consultation room. She was scrolling through my online file that dated back almost 8 years. 'Yeah, but the ones I have are pretty good to me,' I replied.

She smiled and gave me a knowing nod. 'I'll bet!'

I had been in and out of the hospital a number of times over the previous weeks. I was trying hard to get my platelet count high enough for it to be safe to have surgery, and I was waiting to get the go ahead from the blood bank.

My doctor started to look at my maximum platelet levels: how high had I been able to get them in the last 8 years? My highest platelet count on record was 120, which I maintained for one week. Other than the occasional spike and fall, my platelets usually sit between 40-60 (while medicated). At this level, I feel no symptoms and have few problems. I barely notice I even have ITP, and with low medication I'm good to go.

For surgery, I would need to get my platelets much higher - but for regular life, I don't feel the need to push my platelets up that much. It had taken nearly a week of very high doses of prednisone before I had reached a 'normal' range for surgery. But that was not *my* normal range.

For me, it's not about getting back to the 'normal range' anymore. I've forgotten about normal ranges. I have found my own normal and it works well for me. I've told my doctors that a good level for me is 50, and I encourage them not to push for a higher number that can only be achieved through lots of nasty treatments.

I guess this is my acceptance. I would love for my ITP to be gone. But it's hard to get my head around that because I don't like the idea of constantly searching for a more. Instead, happiness now is my highest priority, which oddly enough has seen my platelet count increase.

I have a strange relationship with this stage of ITP. I have felt acceptance a few times over the years, but it didn't last long. When I find myself accepting ITP into my life, I start to worry about what that means. I get nervous that by accepting ITP, I am quitting or giving up. If I accept this, am I saying, 'This is good enough for me?'

Acceptance is hard. It is the precise moment when I am often flung right back to the denial stage. I think about how similar acceptance and denial can be. Am I just in denial that my life is ok? Am I beginning the journey all over again? Have I really made peace with ITP?

I think I have been through each stage three or four times. They are different every time I move through them, but each stage eventually passes to the next one.

I took a long time to define my understanding of acceptance. As a noun, "acceptance" has two different meanings. First, it means to be positively welcomed and accepted by others, and second, to accept something without question. I choose to focus on the first one.

Acceptance is not actually giving up, just giving up the sadness part; accepting that I live with fewer platelets than others and being ok with that.

It doesn't stop. There is more. After almost 8 years with ITP, the craziness is about to start all over again. My husband and I are currently expecting our first full-term ITP baby. As I write this, I am 12 weeks pregnant. We are very excited and eagerly awaiting our next appointment. But will be a very long 9 months. It has already been an enormous 3 months. I can't begin to imagine what the next 6 will be like. I am sure it will definitely be worth all the effort and energy an ITP pregnancy will require.

I will let you know how it goes...

Favorite Things

Websites

Sarahwilson.com

Iquitsugar.com

Paleoforwomen.com

Zenhabits.net

Sproutedkitchen.com

Achievingbalancekinesiology.com.au (Sydney)

Books

Make Peace with Your Plate, by Jess Ainscough

You Can Heal Your Life, by Louise Hay

The Autoimmune Paleo Cookbook, by Mickey Trescott

ITP Blogs

Guide2itp.com

Itpinourwords.blogspot.com.au

Itpsupport.com.au

Katiemeloy.blog.com

Justfrances.com

Rarecandace.com

Missplaquetas.flavors.me

ITP Support

Talking Red'. Talking Red is a new campaign by the Haemophilia Society aimed at getting women talking about bleeding disorders. Bleeding disorders are commonly associated with males, and many people might not know that women can have a bleeding disorder.

The PDSA. The Platelet Disorder Support Association, founded in 1998, is an American non-profit corporation that provides information and support to encourage research about ITP and other platelet disorders. This organisation is devoted to offering the most timely, accurate, and comprehensive information about ITP and platelet disorders.

The ITP Foundation, USA. The ITP Foundation is another American non-profit organization established to raise awareness of Immune Thrombocytopenia. The mission of the ITP Foundation is to increase awareness and help raise funds to further ITP research.

The Australian Centre for Blood Diseases, AUS. This centre aims to provide excellence in the diagnosis and treatment of blood conditions as well as play a leading role in research. The ACBD is involved in research programs, clinical trials and patient education.

The Journal of American Society of Haematology, USA. This is an online and print medical journal. It can appear quite dense and hard to interpret, but there is a great deal of information to be found in this online journal. This is where current research is being published in relation to ITP and other blood disorders.

The ITP Support Association, UK. The ITP Support Association is an independent registered charity which aims to promote and improve the general welfare of people with ITP by providing support and information to patients, their families, and health professionals.

ITP Support, AUS. ITP Support was started in Melbourne as an online resource. It includes online forums, stories and information for ITP patients that is specific to Australia.

Facebook Groups for ITP. There are a number of private ITP groups on Facebook. These groups tend to be divided into regional areas and countries, where patients can share specific information about medical care, local issues and provide more of a community atmosphere.

International ITP Register. Check online for eligibility and criteria. More information can be found at http://itpandme.com/new-international-itp-register-founded-in-australia/.

Terms

Antibodies - An antibody is a large Y-shaped protein that the immune system uses to identify foreign cells and viruses in the body. It is a tag that signals to the immune system that a cell needs to be destroyed.

Arnica - Arnica is a type of flower often used to make medicine. Arnica contains an active ingredient that can be applied to the skin to assist in the pain and swelling of bruises, aches, aprons and insect bites.

Bilirubin - Bilirubin is a by-product of blood breaking down under the skin. Bilirubin is responsible for the brownish yellow colour of bruises as they heal. Bilirubin levels are checked in regular blood samples and an elevated level of bilirubin in the result may be caused by a number of reasons.

Corticosteroids - Corticosteroids are a naturally occurring chemical in the body that includes steroid hormones which are produced by the adrenal cortex. Corticosteroids is a term used for both the naturally occurring hormones in the body and the synthetically manufactured replications of these hormones. Corticosteroids are involved in a wide range of physiological processes including stress, immune response, regulation of inflammation, blood electrolyte levels, and behaviour.

Immunosuppression - A state in which the ability of the body's immune system to respond is decreased. This condition may be present at birth, or it may be caused by certain infections (such as human immunodeficiency virus, HIV). It may also be caused by certain cancer therapies, such as cancer cell killing (cytotoxic) drugs, radiation, and bone marrow transplantation. And from taking corticosteroids.

Intravenous gamma globulin (IVIG) - A man-made protein that contains many antibodies and slows the destruction of platelets; used in the treatment of ITP and other disorders.

NPlate - Also known as romiplostim. The drug romiplostim has been developed by Amgen and is marketed under the trade name NPlate. See below.

Platelet Aggregation - The clumping together of platelets in the blood. Platelet aggregation can also be platelet activation, when the platelet cells grow sticky little arms. Platelet aggregation is part of the sequence of events leading to the formation of a blood clot.

Platelet Counts - Platelets are smaller than red and white blood cells. They are measured in thousands per cubic millimetre of blood (for example 150-400 x 10^9/L). A normal result may vary anywhere from 150,000 - 400,000 platelets per millimetre (mcL).

Rituximab - A treatment available to some ITP patients, depending on their location. Rituximab is classified as chemotherapy, and many countries have not yet approved Rituximab as a mainstream treatment for ITP.

Romiplostim - Also known as NPlate. Romiplostim is a man-made protein medicine designed specifically for patients with ITP. It is used to increase platelet production in the bone marrow by increasing a patient's TPO levels.

Spleen - The spleen is a small organ in your body that is involved in a number of different immune functions. It acts primarily as a blood filter as well as a synthesizer of antibodies in the blood. The removal of the spleen was once a very common treatment of ITP, however, splenectomies have become less popular as they are not always seen as a long-term solution. It is possible to live healthily without a spleen.

TPO Levels - TPO is an acronym for the hormone thyroid peroxidase. This hormone is produced by the thyroid and is stimulated to produce more platelets by the treatment NPlate.

References

1. Alioglu B, Tasar A, Ozen C, Selver B, Dallar Y (2010 November 9) *An experience of oseltamivir phosphate (tamiflu™) in a pediatric patient with chronic idiopathic thrombocytopenic purpura: a case report.* Retrieved from National Centre for Biotechnology http://www.ncbi.nlm.nih.gov/

2. Imbach, P. (2011) Oxidative stress may cause ITP. *Blood.* 117 (17)

3. Ananya, M. (2014 January 14) *What is Oxidative Stress?* Retrieved from http://www.news-medical.net/health

4 / 5. New York Times (1992 September 6) *William J. Harrington, Doctor and Specialist in Blood diseases.* Retrieved from http://www.nytimes.com/

6. Harrington WJ, Minnich V, Hollingsworth JW, Moore CV (1951) *Demonstration of a Thrombocytopenic factor in the blood of Patients with Thrombocytopenic Purpura.* Retrieved from Hematology: Landmark Papers of the Twentieth Century

7. Stasi, R. and Newland, A (2011 May) ITP: A Historical Perspective. *British Journal of Haematology, 153* (4), pages 437–450.

8. Segal JB, Powe NR. J (2006) Prevalence of Immune Thrombocytopenia: Analyses of Administrative Data.

9. Vojdauni, A. (2014) A Potential Link Between Environmental Triggers and Autoimmunity.

10. American Autoimmune Related Diseases Association (2011) The cost burden of Autoimmune Disease: The Latest Front in the War of Healthcare Spending. Retrieved from https://www.aarda.org/

11. The Autoimmune Disease Coordinating Committee (2005) Progress in Autoimmune Diseases Research: National Institutes of Health.

12. Ran, M and Dean, J (2008) Platelet function in autoimmune (idiopathic) thrombocytopenic purpura.

13. Laurence K. Altmen, L K (1986) Who Goes First? The Story of Self-Experimentation in Medicine.

14. Ayesh, M.H. et al. (2013) Adult Primary and Secondary Immune Thrombocytopenic Purpura: A Comparative Analysis of Characteristics and Clinical Course

15. Platelet Disorder Support Association. Retrieved from https://www.pdsa.org/about-itp/inpregnancy.html

16. Gernsheimer, T. James, A. H. and Stasi, R. January 3, 2013; Blood: 121 (1) How I treat thrombocytopenia in pregnancy. Retrieved from http://www.bloodjournal.org/content/121/1/38

17. A Brief History of Traditional Chinese Medicine. Retrieved from http:// www.straighttothepoint.com.au/traditional-chinese-medicine

Thank You

Many thanks to everyone who helped write this book.

Thank you to Alexis Gibson for her close reading and wonderful notes.

Thank you to Leigh for saying yes to every one of my 'ideas'. Thank you to Susie for being my ITP friend.

Thank you to my lovely family for alternatively supporting me and then yelling at me to be healthier in a consistent and loving cycle.

A huge thank you to everyone who continues to read and share through ITP & Me.

Made in the USA
San Bernardino, CA
22 July 2018